Keto Diet

A Complete Guide for Beginners: A Low Carb, High Fat Diet for Weight Loss, Fat Burning and Healthy Living.

By Sarah Maddington

various sources. Please consult a licensed professional before attempting any techniques outlined in this book.

By reading this document, the reader agrees that under no circumstances are is the author responsible for any losses, direct or indirect, which are incurred as a result of the use of information contained within this document, including, but not limited to, —errors, omissions, or inaccuracies.

Table of Contents

Introduction

Many people agree that the ketogenic diet has one of the simplest menus, making it an easy diet to follow. You simply need to eat high-fat, moderate protein, and low-carb foods, which can be easy to get ahold of. By eating a high fat diet, your body will enter a state called ketosis. Ketosis is where your body learns to burn the fat that is already stored, which is why it has weight loss benefits.

Just keep in mind that everyone's body is a little different, so it's important that you pay attention to the signs of ketosis to know when you've entered into it. For many people, it is quick to enter into. Ideally, you'll enter ketosis within a few days, but you'll need to resist the urge to eat high carbs and snack too often.

If you'd like to insure that you enter into ketosis quickly, then you'll want to consider fasting. If you choose not to eat anything containing calories for a full twenty-four hour period, it'll be enough for your body to start breaking down the fat you've stored for energy. However, you'll need to eat a ketogenic friendly meal to keep your body moving forward in its state instead of getting back out of it. Alternatively, if you don't want to fast, then you can just eat ketogenic meals for two to three days, and that should be sufficient to turn your body into a fat burning machine.

The Ketogenic Diet Explained

You already know that the ketogenic diet works by eating high fat with moderate amounts of protein. You'll need to make sure that all of your foods are lwo carb too. It was suspected for a long time that high fat intake resulted in obesity, but in recent years, it has been disproven. Many people over the years have tried and failed to reduce their weight by simply reducing the amount of fat that they eat. However, more sugar was often included in the food. This caused many people to put on weight instead of shedding the pounds they wanted.

Sugar is what resulted in that weight gain. When you eat foods that are high in carbs, the pancreas will create and discharge insulin that makes glucose accessible to platelets. This allows the body to oversee glucose levels, and insluin makes the cells ingest the glucose that's taken from your circulatory system. Without insulin, your cells would not be able todo this. your body will then use the glucose as a primary source of energy, and leftover glucose will then be stored as fat.

If your body has a high amoutn of glucose available to it, it'll burn that instead of your fat stores. This is why ketosis is important. By lowering your carbs, you're lowering the amoutn of glucose your body has to use for energy. This results in ketosis, where your body stops burning the glucose and instead helps you to shed the pounds.

Why the Ketogenic Diet Works for Weight Loss

Many people who start the ketogenic diet find they actually have more energy. This is because your fat works as a wonderful energy source. With this new found energy, you're able to even work out and exercise more, finding more productivity in your daily life. when you get used to exploring healthier but tasty options, you're likely to eat less because you feel sated overall. When you're on the ketogenic diet, you don't count calories. Instead, you count your net carbs. Fat is just as satisfying as protein. this can even help to cut down on cravings.

Some Ketogenic Diet Types

Now that you know how the ketogenic diet can help you to shed the pounds you've wanted, you need to pick which type of ketogenic diet is best for you. There are three mainstream versions of the ketogenic diet. This would be your cyclical ketogenic diet, targeted ketogenic diet, and your standard ketogenic diet.

How can you tell which one is right for you? Look at how fit you currently are and how much exercise you'll be fitting into your routine each week. Most people choose to stick with the standard ketogenic diet, but if you are an athlete, bodybuilder, marathoner or something similar, then you'll want to look at all of your options.

The Standard Ketogenic Diet

This is the diet that most people stick with. It only requires a low amount of physical activity, but it can also work for people who have moderately high levels of exercise. It's the best diet for someone who needs to lose weight and doesn't know where to start. Most people want to at least start with this diet before trying out the other two.

You'll need to follow prescribed amount of carbs, fats and proteins. You'll want to have 80% fat, 15% protein, and only 5% carbs to stay in ketosis. This will also help you to feel like you have an increased amount of energy, but only if you aren't training for a marathon or competitive sport. The energy boost form this type of ketogenic diet is for the standard person.

The Cyclical Ketogenic Diet

This type of ketogenic diet is best if you need to have a day of car bulking before an intense activity. Which is why the cyclical ketogenic diet is best for athletes that are getting ready for a particular event who also have an advanced workout routine. With this type of diet, you're trying to deplete your glycogen stored in your muscles between your workout routines.

You'll still need to use a high-fat and low-carb model most of the time. However, once a week or for two days during each week, you'll eat more carbs. It's best to keep a medium carb intake, but it can include a high carb one. This will let your muscles store the glycogen it needs through the week. If you aren't trying to lose weight, then allow yourself two medium to high carb days each week. The remaining days should be high in fat.

The Targeted Ketogenic Diet

This is the final version of the ketogenic diet, and it requires you to carb bulk right before you start to exercise so that you get the energy boost you need. The goal is that you won't deplete the glycogen stores in your muscles. That's why this type of ketogenic diet is best for elite athletes. Only try this diet if you're a high intensity athlete that works out four to five days each week. This type of ketogenic diet will help to prevent muscle gain or fatigue.

With this type of ketogenic diet, you'll eat a high carb meal once before your workout and within one hour afterwards. The exact amount of carbs you'll need to eat will depend on your normal diet, energy levels, and your body. It can take time to figure out what the right amount is for you.

Some Information Before You Start

It may seem intimidating to start your ketogenic journey, but it doesn't have to be with the right preparation. Yes, it's quite the leap from the standard American diet, but with the right tools and right mentality, you'll be able to stick with the ketogenic diet to meet all of your health goals.

The Right Mindset

Don't let yourself become intimidated or you'll be setting yourself up for failure. The best thing to do is start thinking in the short term instead of the long term. It's important to have long term goals, but if you only focus on the long term everything can easily seem overwhelming. This causes many people to break away from the ketogenic diet before it can even start to help them reach their long term goals. Instead, you'll want to try to set some short term goals that will help you get through your transition period. For example, stop telling yourself that you'll never be able to eat carbs again. At the beginning, this will seem like an impossible feat. Instead, tell yourself that you're going to take a break from carbs for a certain amount of time, such as week or a month. Commit to that set of time, and then allow yourself your first cheat day. If you stick to your goal, knowing you'll be able to cheat afterwards, then you're more likely to achieve that goal. You'll also need to get used to the idea that you will have cravings, and this is a completely natural part of any diet. At some point during your first month, you're going to start craving carbs, but you don't actually need them. To overcome your cravings, remind yourself that overtime they'll lose their intensity and that you will eventually have a cheat day.

Prepare the Kitchen

Preparing your kitchen is an essential part of going keto. Most people have tons of processed foods, pasta and bread in their kitchen. If you have them on hand, it'll be harder to keep from giving into your cravings. Once you've committed to the ketogenic diet, get rid of these foods so that they don't tempt you! If you have a family that doesn't want to commit to the keto lifestyle, then try keeping a cabinet that's full of your ketogenic foods so that they're separate from the food that triggers cravings. It'll be up to you to keep away from the cabinets and drawers that hold temptation.

When you're just starting the ketogenic diet you, you'll want to keep the food simple. Don't try to make fancy ketogenic recipes like grain-free bread or crackers. You may want to stay away from keto dessert to. Instead, fill your kitchen with fresh vegetables, ketogenic approved cheese, and ketogenic fruit. You'll need to buy plenty of eggs and various meats. Concentrate on learning how to make some simple and quick keto meals so that you always have something to eat in a pinch.

Prepare for the First Few Weeks

These first weeks are going to be the hardest, but they're crucial to your success too. You're going to go through various changes in the first few weeks. You're certain to lose weight, but eventually you'll hit a plateau. Mood swings, especially anger, will be common. It's natural to feel hungry and tired at first, and as with any diet, you're likely going to get frustrated. Having a clear expectation of what will happen before you make progress is an important step in sticking with the ketogenic lifestyle.

About The Keto Flu

This is a nickname for some physical changes you'll go through when you first get rid of the carbs. Your body is going without something that it's started to feel is essential, so it's normal for it to react poorly. That's where the headaches, nausea, fatigue and other uncomfortable reactions come into play, aka the keto flu.
Not everyone experiences this, but most people do. The intensity varies from person to person, and it's likely you'll have a foggy mind for a while. If you want to avoid the ketogenic flu, then you'll need to introduce the keto diet quickly. Slowly reduce the carbs you consume for four to six

weeks before committing to the keto lifestyle. If you want to jump right in, you'll get over it faster. No matter what you do, try increasing your intake of salt and fluid. Drinking a few cups of bouillon can do wonders at reducing the symptoms. Don't panic, know that's it normal, and power through it to gain all of the benefits that come with the keto diet.

Take Control of Your Sugar Cravings

There's no escaping the sugar cravings that are bound to happen when you first start the keto diet. They'll hit even harder when you're hungry or in need of a snack. Your first thoughts will likely be cookies, cakes or bread of some kind. Don't fear! There are ways to beat the cravings. The best tip is to stay prepared. Try to recognize the times that you're usually hungry, and make sure that you have keto approved snacks on hand. Carrots, low car peanut butter, dark chocolate or unprocessed cheeses can help. It'll prevent you from giving in and heading to the nearest vending machine to satisfy your cravings for carbs.

The Start of Weight Loss

After the first week of the keto diet, many people will experience a drop in their body weight. This can be motivating and exciting for many people, but it's important to be realistic. At this time, most of the weight you're losing is water weight and excess carbs that were stored in your body. Eventually, your weight loss will slow down and you'll hit a plateau. Try not to get bummed out! Just stick with the ketogenic diet, and eventually the pounds will once again start to melt away. Usually you'll start experiencing weight loss again in sixty to ninety days.

The Takeaway

The most important thing to prepare for the ketogenic diet is your mind and your kitchen. When you're mentally prepared for the hardships you'll face, it'll be easier to stay committed during the first few weeks of your new keto lifestyle. It's even easier when you've prepared your pantry to remove all the tempting foods you were used to eating, which in turn will increase your chance of success!

Ketogenic Diet Essentials

In this diet, you'll learn some ketogenic diet essentials that will help you to reach all of your weight loss goals!

Some Terms & Knowledge

In this book, carbohydrates, as I'm sure you've already noticed, will often be called carps for short. Ketosis, which is also known as nutritional ketosis, refers to how many ketones are in your blood, and the ketogenic diet will often, as you've seen, be referred to as the keto diet. The keto diet is a way to lose weight while lessening your risk of disease. It gives you good food that will sate you so that hunger pangs are a thing of the past. Many people lose double the amoutn of weight on the ketogenic diet as they do on many low-fat diets.

About Ketogenesis

This is a biochemical process in which your body will produce large amounts of ketones, which cause the breakdown of fatty acids. It'll also break down the ketogenic amino acids in your liver.

In Reference to Weight loss

The keto diet is famous for helping in weight loss, and it's been sued by celebrities and athletes worldwide. With the keto diet, anyone can reach the state of ketosis, turning their body into a fat burning machine.

Ketosis vs. Ketoacidosis

The first thing you need to know is that ketosis is a controlled process, and ketoacidosis is not. That's why ketosis is safe and ketoacidosis isn't. In ketosis, your body regulates your insulin. Ketoacidosis does not, making it an unhealthy state of being.

Some Basic Principles

Here are some basic principles before you start preparing healthy, tasty keto food.

Simple Principles

There are a few principles you'll need to adhere to if you want to start your keto diet.

- **The 60-75% Rule:** Keep this percentage for your fat, and 15-30% for protein, and 5-10% for carbs.
- **Net Carbs:** You'll need to pay attention to your net carb consumption too. Make sure it doesn't exceed fifty grams. If you need to calculate your net carbs, then take the total carbs minus the dietary fiber and minus the sugar to equal your net carbs.
- **Moderate Proteins:** Don't oversaturate your diet with proteins either if you want the keto diet to work for you. You'll need to take your current body fat percentage to determine the amount of protein you should be eating you should choose between 0.6-1 gram per pound of lean body mass.
- **The Proper Fats:** Make sure that your calories from fat come from standard types such as omega-3s, monounsaturated fats and saturated fats.
- **Avoid Most Fruits:** You'll need to avoid most fruits and low carb treats to keep your net carb low.

- **Never Starve:** You should never starve yourself. Eat when you're hungry and just calculate your net carbs to lose the weight you want.

- **Never Ignore Your Body:** While it's important to keep your net carbs and calorie intake low, never ignore when you're hungry or you'll end up falling off the ladder.

- **Stock Up:** You'll need to stock up on keto friendly foods such as non-starchy vegetables, eggs, coconut oil, meat, macadamia nuts, bone broth, avocados, and fermented foods.

- **Avoid Processed Fats:** Processed fats are bad news for your diet, so avoid vegetable oils, partially hydrogenated oils, fully hydrogenated oils, trans fat, soybean oil, corn oil, canola oil and trans fat.

- **Eat Raw & Organic:** You'll need to eat organic and raw dairy products if you don't have any allergies. Though, try to avoid milk due to the high carb content.

- **Increase Your Electrolytes:** Increase your intake of electrolytes because the keto diet may cause sodium, potassium and calcium deficiency. It's also important to increase your salmon, avocados, mushrooms, nut, and magnesium supplements, salt and bone broth.

- **Avoid Processed Foods:** Many processed foods have hidden carbs such as preservatives, additives, artificial sweeteners, sorbitol, and maltitol, which means you should avoid them all together.

- **Ignore Certain Labels:** Foods with labels such as fat-free, low fat or low carb usually contain artificial additives and extra carbs in their ingredient list. It's best to avoid them.

- **Check Your Medication:** Some medications contain sweeteners or sugars, so try to get the sugar free varieties.

- **Plan Ahead:** It's best to plan ahead so that you avoid spontaneous eating which will ruin your diet.

- **Shop Weekly:** You'll need to shop frequently in order to keep the right ingredients on hand.

- **Hard Boiled Eggs:** Hard boiled eggs and salads make a great easy keto friendly snack when you're in a pinch!

Benefits to Keep in Mind

You already know that the keto diet can help you to shed those unwanted pounds, but there are other benefits too!

Improved Focus

One lovely perk of the keto diet is an improved focus and concentration. Once you reach a state of ketosis, your brain is getting a constant flow of ketones. Even if you're already physically fit, the keto diet can help to improve your mental performance. The best part is that this diet doesn't allow your blood sugar levels to go up and down too much.
It's a common misconception that higher brain functions require a lot of carbs. This is only true if you don't have ketones available. Give your body a week, and it'll function smoothly on ketones. You'll only get this perk once you get over the keto flu.

Physical Endurance

the keto diet can help with your physical endurance as well as your mental focus. The glycogen your body stores can only last for a few hours of activities, but your fat reserves have enough energy to last quite some time. It can last for weeks or even months. Since your body is used to relying on carbs for energy, it isn't tapping into your fat reserves even if it's for your brain. This requires you to eat during, after or even before a workout to avoid hunger pangs. The keto diet will help you to avoid this drawback.

Lowered Cholesterol

The keto diet also helps to improve your triglyceride and cholesterol levels too. It'll increase your HDL, which is considered your good cholesterol, and lower your LDL which is your bad cholesterol. This can help anyone, but it's particularly useful for someone who's having cholesterol issues. It can also lower your risk of heart disease.

Type 2 Diabetes Treatment

Since the keto diet is a low carb diet, it helps many people to reverse type 2 diabetes. The main cause of type 2 diabetes is high blood sugar. The sugar results from the carbs you consume, and so the less sugar you eat means the less sugar that's in your blood. In turn, this lowers your blood sugar level. It's normal for the keto diet to dramatically drop your blood sugar levels to a normal rate. If you're suffering from type 2 diabetes, then you'll need to talk to your doctor before starting the keto diet. If you are already taking a medication to drop your blood sugar, then the dosage might need to be decreased to keep your blood sugar from dropping dangerously. The keto diet can help with type 1 diabetes as well, but it will not reverse it.

Foods to Start With

As you shed the pounds, you're still going to need to eat. You just have to know what you can and can't eat if you want to stick to the keto lifestyle.

Fats & Oils

The majority of your calorie intake will be fats, so it's important to make sure that you're consuming the right fat. There are different ways that you can add fat to your meal. It can be in sauces, dressing, or simply as a topping on a piece of meat, including butter. Fat is vital to your body, and below you'll find the right type of fat for your diet.

- **Saturated Fats:** Some examples of saturated fats are ghee, coconut oil, butter and lard.
- **Monounsaturated Fats:** Some examples of monounsaturated fats are olive, avocado, and macadamia nut oils.
- **Polyunsaturated Fats:** You need to know the difference. There are naturally polyunsaturated fats such as fatty fish or animal proteins which are healthy to eat. However, if it isn't a naturally occurring polyunsaturated fat, such as a margarine saying its heart healthy, isn't something you should be eating.

Below you'll find the fat you should always avoid.

- **Trans Fat:** You need to completely avoid this type of fat. This type of fat has been chemically altered to have a longer shelf life and can lead to heart disease.

You'll also want to balance your omega-6s and omega-3s. If you don't like fish, you'll want to try an omega-3 supplement. Omega-3's are great for you and can be found in wild salmon, trout, shellfish, and even tuna. However, seed or nut based foods can be high in omega-6s which are inflammatory. These include pine nuts, sunflower oil, corn oil, almonds and walnuts. You'll need to keep these items balanced if you don't want to have an inflammation problem. Essential fatty acids provide your body with what it needs for core function.

Below you'll find some healthy oils you should try.

- Brazil Nuts/Macadamia
- Butter/Ghee
- Coconut Butter
- Fatty fish
- Non-hydrogenated Animal Fat
- Tallow
- Avocados
- Lard
- Egg Yolks
- Coconut Oil
- Cocoa Butter
- Olive Oil
- Macadamia Oil
- MCT Oil

- Avocado Oil

Eat Your Protein

There are many protein sources that you can have on the keto diet. However, the high amount of protein, the less you should consume. It's better to stick with grass-fed and pasture-raised protein if you can. This will help to minimize your steroid hormone intake and bacteria intake. Try to choose darker meats when dealing with poultry, as it's much fattier than white meat. Eating fatty fish is also great. When you're dealing with red meat, there isn't much you need to worry about avoiding. Just try to avoid cured meats and sausages because they often have added processed ingredients and sugar. If you're eating steak, try to choose a fattier cut. If you want ground beef, choose a fattier ratio too. Just be careful of your protein intake. Too much protein means lower levels of ketones, which will increase your glucose production which will take you right out of ketosis. You'll go back to burning glucose instead of burning fat. Try to balance out your protein with fatty sauces and side dishes. If you're choosing to eat lean beef, you need to be even more careful with portion control.

Here are some meats to eat.

- **Fish:** Try to eat fish that's been caught wild, such as flounder, halibut, mackerel, catfish, cod, mahi-mahi, salmon, trout, tuna and snapper. The fattier the fish the better.

- **Shellfish:** Lobster, crab, mussels, scallops, squid, oysters and clams are great for the keto diet.
- **Beef:** Try roasts, steak, ground beef, and stew meat. The fattier the cuts the better.
- **Pork:** Ground pork, pork chops, pork loin, tenderloin and ham are great. Just watch out for added sugar in pork items, and make sure you choose fatty cuts.
- **Whole Eggs:** Free-range eggs are great, especially if you can get them from a local market. The best part is that they're versatile, so you can eat them scrambled, poaches, fried, boiled or deviled.
- **Offal/Organ:** There are many organs that are great to eat such as tongue, heart, kidney and liver. These organs are a great source of nutrients and vitamins.
- **Nut Butters:** Go for a natural nut butter, so common peanut butter usually isn't good enough. Make sure that they're unsweetened. You can even make your own. Since legumes, such as peanuts, are high in omega-6s it's best to avoid it whenever possible.
- **Poultry:** Try wild game, chicken, quall, pheasant and duck.
- **Bacon & Sausage:** If you're going to eat sausage or bacon, then check labels to see if it's cured or has sugar. You also need to watch out for fillers, but you shouldn't be too concerned with nitrates.
- **Other Meat:** Try lamb, turkey, wild game, goat, or veal. Just stick with fatty cuts when you can.

Fruit & Vegetables

There are some do's and don'ts when it comes to vegetables and fruits that are ketogenic friendly. Vegetables are important to the keto diet, but some still need to be avoided because they're too high in sugar or starch. You need vegetables that are low in carbs and high in nutrients. It's best to stick with dark and leafy. Try to eat cruciferous vegetables which are leafy, green and above ground. This includes spinach, kale, cabbage and more. They are great if they're frozen or fresh. You can still consume vegetable that grow below ground in moderation, but you need to be aware of the amount of carbs they have.

Watch out for the vegetable groups below.

- **Nightshades:** Some nightshades to avoid are peppers, tomato and eggplant.
- **Berries:** Sadly, berries aren't very keto friendly either, including blueberries, raspberries or blackberries.
- **Citrus:** Lemon, lime, and oranges aren't great for the keto diet. This includes their juice or zest.
- **Root Vegetables:** Onion, garlic, mushrooms, squash, and parsnip are bad for you too. Try to stay away from root vegetables in general.

You'll need to completely avoid large fruits like bananas and potatoes too.

A Look at Dairy

The higher the amount of carbs in the dairy products, the less you'll want to consume if you're trying to stick to the ketogenic lifestyle. Just try to keep your dairy consumption moderate. If you can, try to eat raw and organic dairy products. Always choose full fat products over a low fat or fat free alternative. Low fat and fat free options aren't filling and yet are high in carbs.

If you're sensitive to lactose, then try to have long-aged dairy products that have less lactose but are still keto. You'll find some options below.

- Cottage Cheese
- Cream Cheese
- Sour Cream
- Crème Fraiche
- Mascarpone
- Aged Cheddar
- Parmesan Cheese
- Feta Cheese
- Swiss Cheese
- Heavy Whipping Cream
- Greek Yogurt
- Homemade Mayonnaise

When you add dairy, you're adding extra fat to a meal. You can also create creamy side dishes such as spinach, and it's a great way to add a sauce too.

Seeds & Nuts

Nuts and seeds are great on the keto diet, but they're even better if they're roasted so that you remove any anti-nutrients. Just try to avoid peanuts if you can since they're a legume, which aren't keto friendly. Typically, adding in raw nuts can add texture or flavor to your meal. Some people even choose them as a snack, but that isn't weight loss friendly. Snacking will raise insulin levels, so avoid it if you can.

Raised insulin means slower weight loss. However, nuts are a great way to get fats, but they do have a carb count that can add up quickly. They even contain protein that you need to watch out for. Try to avoid nut flours since they will add protein fast. They're also high in omega-6 fatty acids, which you need to limit the consumption of. You'll find a list of nuts broken down and how they'll affect you below.

- **Low Carb & Fatty Nuts:** Brazil nuts, pecans, and macadamia nuts.
- **Moderate Carbs & Fatty Nuts:** Almonds, hazelnuts, walnuts, pine nuts and peanuts.
- **High Carb Nuts:** Cashews and pistachios should be avoided.

You'll likely use nut and seed flours when you need to substitute regular flour, but you still need to be careful. Though, they're often used in keto desserts.

Sweeteners

Just because you're on the keto diet doesn't mean you need to give up everything sweet. Just try to go with sweeteners that have a small amount of sugar count, such as stevia, cleric essential item, Splenda, Sweet n Low, and others like this. It's best to go with the liquid version if possible since they don't have binders that could work against you.

Side Effects & How to Avoid Them

Every diet can have side effects if you don't start it properly, but with this chapter you'll learn the risks of the keto diet and how to avoid them. You already know that the keto flu is a major downside and how to get over it, so let's get acquainted with a few other possibilities.

Bad breath

When you're just getting started with the keto diet, or a low carb diet in general, you'll find that bad breath is a risk. This comes from the acetone, which is a type of ketone. It can smell like nail polish remember or just bad breath. It can also be a body odor that lasts from not staying hydrated enough, or just odor from exercising more. You may need to kick up the showers and mouthwash a little to avoid this downside.

Some people don't experience this symptom. For those who do, it's often temporary. It should disappear when you become adapted to your diet. Drinking more water can usually help with this, as a dry mouth means that the bacteria in your mouth isn't getting cleaned away by your saliva. This can lead to severe breath, so staying hydrated will serve a double purpose!

Leg cramps

It's normal to deal with leg cramps at the start of your new ketogenic lifestyle. Though they don't usually cause a serious issue they can be painful. This is due to the loss of magnesium and an increase of urination. Sat and water when mixed together can make a good drink once a day to keep you retaining more water, resulting in less magnesium being loss. However, many people find that a magnesium supplement works better. Only eat more carbs as a last resort since it'll weaken the effects of your keto diet.

Higher Cholesterol

The keto diet encourages you to consume foods that are high in fat. Most of the time, you'll find that the keto diet is great at evening out or even improving your cholesterol, but there is trouble around the corner for some. Some people find that their good cholesterol starts to exceed the average level, which can be a problem in itself. If you're having this issue, then lower your fat intake a little.

Do not increase your protein intake. If you aren't feeling hungry, just try to eat less net carbs a day. You can also drink things that are lower in fat content. Intermittent fasting can be a solution as well, but it'll only work for a short period. Trying to concentrate on getting the fats you need for unsaturated fat can be a big help to lower your cholesterol too. It can also help to prevent stroke and heart disease. Try adding more olive oil, avocados or fatty fish into your diet.

Easy Intoxication

When you start the keto diet, you'll find that you become intoxicated easily. It is suspected that it is due to the liver busily creating ketones, so it doesn't digest the liquor quite as fast as others. When you start your keto lifestyle, just be prepared for a lower alcohol tolerance. You should also be aware of how many carbs alcoholic drinks really contain, which will pull you out of ketosis.

Choose your drinks wisely. If you want a cocktail, try a Bloody Mary, since it only has seven net carbs. A margarita has eight net carbs, and a cosmopolitan has thirteen grams! However, not every drink is prepared the same, so make sure that you're getting exactly what you want. Champagne is a great choice since it usually only has one gram per serving. Just know what you're drinking adjust your day's meal plan accordingly.

Enduring the Keto Rash

Some people experience a rash when they get started with the keto diet, but as your body adjusts it will naturally start to go away. In the meantime, try to wear comfortable clothing that's appropriate for your weather. You may also want to adjust your exercise program so that you have time to shower to get the sweat from your skin. Some people are lucky enough not to experience the keto rash at all.

Some More Drawbacks

Like with every diet, there are drawbacks, and you'll find them laid out for you below.

- **Low Energy:** While the keto diet can help to increase your energy levels after a while, you'll find that it actually decreases them at first.
- **Food Restrictions:** Just like with every diet, there are things you can't eat. You'll need to give these foods up if you want a chance at success.
- **Metabolic Problems:** You'll need to pay attention to your metabolic function because a low carb diet for extended periods of time can decrease your metabolic function if not monitored.

The Keto Diet & Your Metabolism

Many critics of the ketogenic diet often say it messes with your metabolism, but is this really true? To understand the answer, you need to understand what your metabolism actually does. Your metabolism primarily makes fuel for your body when it's needed. As you continue to eat food, your metabolic system will make sure that your body uses the foods properly.

It will then store the excess as fat.

When you eat too much, then your metabolic system has more to cope with than it was actually designed to handle. During the starvation, your system focuses on providing glucose where it needs to be. It's usually gotten from the muscles, but it can also be pulled from the fat. Since your metabolic system doesn't know how long you'll starve, it'll plunder your glucose supply form your muscles.

However, it doesn't want to your muscle mass to be depleted, so it'll look to ketones for a solution. Ketones can stand in for proteins and glucose, so your muscles won't need to be depleted. Your body happily uses these ketones as a source of fuel and general energy. Now, since you're on a low carb diet instead of a starvation diet, you'll also be taking in proteins and fats which will also help to keep your muscles from being depleted. The proteins you eat will be converted to glucose.

Now, back to the question. Will the ketogenic diet ruin your metabolism? The metabolism isn't completely dependent on what you do or don't eat. There is the basal metabolic rate, which is dependent on your lean body mass, genetic tendencies and homeostasis. Any diet at all would affect this type of metabolic rate.

You also have to keep in mind the thermic effect of food, which is an energy that breaks down the macronutrients from the food you consume so that your body can process them. Protein is the highest amount of energy, but low carb diets improve the metabolism.

The thermic effect of activity also needs to be considered. Any form of activity that isn't a necessary body function such as exercise is included in this. If you are sedentary or inactive, then you'll burn less energy, so your metabolism is less. So, the ketogenic diet cannot truly destroy your metabolism. No matter what diet you're on, it won't actually destroy your metabolism unless you are completing starving yourself and refusing physical activity.

A Quick Reminder

The keto diet isn't a miracle weight loss solution, and it's certainly not a yo-yo diet. It's a lifestyle change, and you have to have the discipline needed to stay on it. It is hard work, but you can adjust to it. You also can't expect this diet to work without at least moderate exercise. For better weight loss results, you're going to want to have more frequent exercise or even more intense exercise.

Debunking Some Ketogenic Diet Myths

Like with any diet, there are some myths surrounding it. You need all the facts before you decide to commit to a lifestyle change, and that's what this chapter is about.

You Need Carbs to Have a Healthy Body

Even though carbs are a great source of energy, they are not the only source of energy. Therefore, you don't need carbs to be healthy. The brain needs glucose from carbs to function, and this is true. However, the lack of carbs will not keep your brain from functioning. As soon as you enter ketosis, your body takes on a glucose sparing effect. Once it's adjusted to the ketogenic diet, then it can fuel with ketones instead of glucose and still be healthy.

Ketosis is Dangerous.

Too much of anything can be dangerous, but this doesn't mean ketosis is bad for you. This is where it is essential to understand the difference between ketoacidosis, which is harmful, from ketosis, which is fine. The ketogenic diet will result in ketosis not ketoacidosis.

Ketones Can Damage Your Kidneys

This is based on a misunderstanding. Your kidneys can be damaged if you eat too much protein. However, the keto diet concentrates on high fat instead of high protein. Though, eating a small amount of protein that isn't necessary won't be enough to actually hurt you. So even some high protein days won't cause any damage.

It'll Clog Your Arteries

Since people on the keto diet consume a large amount of fat, then it's normal to think it'll clog your arteries and lead to heart disease. Though, this isn't the case. The keto diet won't just let you eat any fat you want. You still only need to consume healthy fats that come with good cholesterol. Cholesterol itself isn't necessarily bad. Your cells need it, but there is a good and bad type. That's why the keto diet doesn't lead to your arteries being clogged.

It's Bad For Your Colon

This is another myth that's completely wrong. The keto diet does include food that has all the fiber you need, such as cabbage, spinach and many others. This means, the keto diet is actually good for your colon. Many people that use the keto diet actually have a healthier colon than before, and they're often more regular as a result.

Your Muscles Will Shrink

This myth isn't true because ketones are available, so you won't be depleting your muscles. It's also important to note that the keto diet does encourage you to eat enough proteins on a daily basis that you don't lose any muscle mass at all.

It'll Make Your Body Weak

This is yet another myth about the keto diet that simply isn't true. You'll experience improved physical and mental performance after you get over the keto flu. You may feel weak the start, but that will change once your body has released ketones and you actually enter ketosis.

Entering & Measuring Ketosis

To be in ketosis, your serum ketones need to be between 0.5-30 M. You really don't' have to measure your ketones to have keto diet success. If you stick to the diet properly, you're going to enter it. However, everyone does this at different rates. If you are curious, though, there are different things you can do to measure your ketosis properly.

Blood Ketone Meter

This is an exact way to quantify your beta-hydroxybutyrate. It can decide with accuracy the level of ketones in your blood. Though, they're costly. Most meters will cost $40 and the strips cost $5. However, if you're trying to gauge your levels on a daily basis, you'll need about $150.

Urine Ketone Strips

Your urine can demonstrate an overabundance of ketones in the body, which will be discharged as urine. That makes this type of test to be accurate. Though, they can be tough to find and still cost a good penny.

Perception

Despite the tests on the market, many people will choose to just stay in tune with their body. You'll have a "fruity" odor in your sweet, breath, and urine when you first start ketosis. If you pick up on this, it's likely you're already in ketosis.

Common Keto Diet Mistakes

There are mistakes in any new diet, and they can surely hamper your success. However, if you have an idea of what common mistakes that can be made, then you are able to avoid them a little easier.

Cool the Pressure Down

It's important that you chop down your pressure if you want to lose weight properly. You can't expect to speed through this diet. That expectation will cause you to fail. You need to be realistic about what you'll achieve, and you need to choose goals that are realistic as well.

Eating Prepared Food

This is another simple mistake that far too many people make. When you're eating foods that have already been prepared, then they're not using the freshest ingredients. They likely have fillers and hidden sugars as well that will sabotage your goals.

Not Staying Focused

If you don't stay focused, then you're sure to fall short of your goals. Most weight watchers that don't put their diet first, will never lose the weight they want. You need to count your net carbs and plan your meals in advance. If you don't do that, you will fail.

Comparing Yourself to Others

If you're constantly comparing your body to someone else's, then you're damaging your ability to see your successes. Everyone's body is different, so everyone will react to the keto diet at different weights. Your friend may go on the keto diet with you, but they may lose weight faster. That's normal. You just have to take it one day at a time.

Not Taking Vitamins

The ketone diet may mean that you're consuming less calories, but it's important that you keep your vitamins up. A multivitamin can come a long way in keeping you healthy while you switch over to ketosis. Feeling as best as you can while you transition will keep your body ready for the long haul.

Eating the Wrong Fats

You can't just eat any greasy food that you want. As stated before, only the right types of fat will help you. With the wrong types of fats, you'll only end up hurting your health and weight loss goals. make sure you understand the type of fat your'e consuming during the day.

Eating Too Little

If you're counting your calories too much, then you're not doing it right. You need to manage your hunger, and eating too little can hinder your weight loss goals too. Many people that try to use the keto diet try to cut down their calories too much when all they should really be watching is their net carbs.

Eating too Many Carbs

If you consume too many carbs, then you're not going to stay in ketosis. If you weigh 150 pounds, then you should only have thirty grams of net carbs. On the keto diet, it's best to stick with 20 net carbs each day.

Eating Too Little Fat

If you eat too little fat, then your body won't have what it needs to function. Just like your body will have too low of energy without starches, your fat takes the place, giving you the energy you need. If you cut out the fat too, then you're going to end up exhausted and feeling ill.

Getting the Most Out of Your Diet

To get the best results in the shortest amount of time, then follow these ketogenic diet tips!

Read the Labels

While as a rule of thumb, it's best to avoid something that has a nutrition label since it isn't a whole food. Though, it's actually hard to avoid. You're eventually going to use something that's prepared. Look at the serving size. If it says one package as the serving, then you can check the rest. If it says two per package, then remember that you'll need to divide in half. Anything but one serving, means you need to divide by that number. The label should outline proteins, carbs and fat. It should also tell you about sugars and dietary fibers, which means you can calculate your net carbs. You should also check to see if it has Trans or hydrogenated fats, and if so then you can avoid it.

Sleeping & Ketosis

When people first start ketosis, it's not uncommon for them to suffer from a bout of insomnia. This happens because your body is still learning to adapt without carbs. Carbs are a source of tryptophan, which helps you to relax for sleep. Without this, your body has a hard time getting to rest at night. You can offset this by taking a tryptophan supplement. Though, over time your body will get used to it even without the supplement. It can also help if you implement high levels of exercise.

Stay Hydrated

It's common to forget to hydrate effectively, but it becomes even more important if you're on a new diet. Your body won't function properly if you aren't getting enough water in the day. You can drink tea, keto coffee, keto smoothies and water on the keto diet, which will help you to stay hydrated during the day.

Exercise in Intervals

It's important to exercise in intervals too if you want the best results! You'll want to try to exercise at least twenty to thirty minutes every day so that you can get into a routine. You'll also want to alternate what type of exercise you use. It's easy to squeeze in twenty minutes a day, especially if you remind yourself that it's essential to your goals.

Manage Your Stress

Stress can cause people to fall off the wagon with anything, and the ketogenic diet is no different. Try to find a little time for you every single day. Meditation, yoga, or even just reading for thirty minutes can help. Stress hormones elevate blood sugar, which will work against your keto diet.

Ketogenic Diet Q&A

You're almost ready to start your keto journey, but let's go through some common question and answers before you begin cooking some keto friendly meals.

Do I have to count calories?

The truth is no, you don't. Over the long term, you won't need to count calories to stay on the right track. Your body will burn the energy, and you won't deal with glucose spikes that cause weight gain. High fat foods will help you to feel sated and stay that way for longer periods of time. Naturally, you'll start to eat less.

What snacks can I have?

It's best to avoid snacking as much as you can, but this isn't easy for everyone. Various nuts, seeds, and keto friendly cheeses can be used as long as you count the net carbs. You'll also want to try fresh vegetables and homemade nut butters whenever you can. There are many ketogenic snacks out there that you can prepare in advance too. You can even make ketogenic sweets.

Can I cheat on the keto diet?

Yes, you can eventually have cheat days. Though, when you're just starting, you'll want to commit 100% committed to your diet. You have to get your body adapted to the keto diet before you start allowing yourself to cheat every now and then. The more you get used to your new lifestyle, the less you'll feel the need to cheat your diet.

Do I really go into starvation mode?

No, that's a common myth. You won't be starving, but you may be hungry if you're counting your net carbs and calories at first. You'll get used to it though.

Can I combine this diet with others?

Its best not to combine the keto diet with another diet because it can cause the keto diet to mess up. It can also cause you to get sick, so try to only stick to one diet at a time. Though, many people view the keto diet as a lifestyle choice.

Can the keto diet be vegan or vegetarian?

Since those are also a lifestyle choice and not just a diet, yes, you can safely pair the keto diet with veganism or vegetarianism. However, you may need to talk to your doctor to make sure that you aren't missing any vital nutrients or vitamins by doing so.

Tips for Eating Out

Just because you're committing to the keto diet, doesn't mean that you can't eat out. You'll just need to be a little more careful about it, which is what this chapter will help you with.

Start with Research

You'll need to research where you're going if possible. Once you get used to eating out on the keto diet, you can go to spur of the moment food events, but this won't always be the case. You should see which diets are gluten free, for example, as it pairs well with keto. You can also check their menus before you go. See if there is anything on the menu that is carb free before going somewhere.

Call Them

Try calling them to see if they are equipped to cater to someone on a low carb diet. If they say yes, you can ask what choices they have available. You may only find they have one or two options, but that can be enough to go out and enjoy a night with friends and family.

Avoid Temptation

You'll want to avoid restaurants that have too many high carb ingredients. If they liter every meal, then you're likely to want to cheat on the keto diet, which can push all of your goals back. It can also help to pick out your meal before you go, so you know exactly what you want to order and won't be tempted by anything else. It's easier to fight the temptation when it won't be delivered to you immediately after thinking it looks good, so try to fight it at home to make the right decision.

Double Check Everything

You can never be too careful when you decide to eat prepared food rather than make it yourself. If you're served a meal that has something on it you can't have and you asked to be removed, send it back. Don't try to pick around it. There's no reason for the temptation to be there.

Avoid Appetizers

It's usually best you avoid appetizers when you're trying to eat healthy. Appetizers are loaded with extra calories and oil, and usually they're loaded with unhealthy fats too. Remember that you have a limited amount of net carbs you're allowed, so don't waste it on an appetizer.

Ask Questions

You can always ask your waiter or waitress if something can be substituted. Maybe you can get that hamburger wrapped in lettuce instead of the bun, for example. Then you can pair it with a side salad, and you'll be good to go. You can also take out sauces that aren't healthy for you if they're the only thing in the dish that's bad for you. You may want to ask them about what certain dishes or components are made from too.

Avoid Most Drinks

Don't order cocktails or mocktails. You need to be careful with tea or coffee to. Your drink choice will matter when you're counting your net carbs. Drinks will rack up net carbs and bring you out of ketosis, especially because they won't actually fill you up or keep you full.

Remember Your Portions

Try to remember that the portions that you eat when you're at a restaurant is usually more than you should be having at a meal. They're usually bigger than the portions that you'd have at home too. If you've already been served a big portion, try to just pack some home to take for later. You may want to ask for something to pack the rest of it up before you get your plate, so that you only have what you plan to eat in front of you. This will keep you from overeating and ruining your state of ketosis.

Look at How It's Cooked

Your entrees are where most of your net carbs and calories will come for. It's important to figure out how the meat is being prepared. It's best to go with something that's poached, broiled, sautéed, grilled, steamed or baked if you want to go with the healthy choice. It's best if there's no oil.

Control Your Sweet Cravings

Dessert is a huge issue when you're eating out. There are very few low carb desserts, and remember the dangers of low fat food when you're on the keto diet. So, check in advance if there is anything in the dessert section that you can eat. You may want to choose something form the kids food menu too. You may just want to get that glass of sweet tea for dessert, since it'll be less damaging than an actual dessert on the menu.

Recipes to Get You Started

Now you know everything you need to about the ketogenic diet to get you started on your ketogenic journey. Here are a few recipes that you can start with to help you reach your weight loss goals without sacrificing taste.

Buttery Green Eggs

Serves: 2
Time: 20 Minutes
Ingredients:
- 2 Tablespoons Butter
- ½ Cup Cilantro, Fresh & Chopped
- 4 Eggs
- 1 Teaspoon Thyme, Fresh & Chopped
- 1 Tablespoon Coconut Oil
- ½ Cup Parsley, Fresh & Chopped
- 2 Cloves Garlic, Peeled & chopped
- ¼ Teaspoon Cumin
- ¼ Teaspoon Cayenne
- ½ Teaspoon Sea Salt, Fine

Directions:
1. Let your coconut oil and butter together for sixty seconds, and then add in your garlic. Cook for three minutes on low. Your garlic should become fragrant and brown.
2. Add your thyme, allowing it to brown which will take about half a minute. Make sure you don't let it burn.
3. Add your cilantro and parsley, turning your heat to medium. They should become crispy.
4. Add in your eggs, but be careful not to break the yolk.
5. Cover your pan before reducing your heat to low.
6. Cook for five to six minutes. Your yolks should still be soften, and serve warm.

Nutrition Facts:
Calories: 311

Fat: 27.5 Grams
Net Carbs: 2.5 Grams
Protein: 12.8 Grams

Easy Spinach Omelet

Serves: 2
Time: 25 Minutes
Ingredients:

- 1 Cup Spinach, Fresh & Chopped
- 1 Cup Swiss Chard, Fresh & Chopped
- 3 Eggs
- 2 Cloves Garlic, Crushed
- 2 Tablespoons Olive Oil
- 1 Teaspoon Celery, Dried
- ½ Teaspoon Sea Salt, Fine
- ¼ Teaspoon Red Pepper Flakes

Directions:

1. Start by rinsing your greens under cold water, and then drain in a colander before setting it to the side.
2. Grease your skillet with your olive oil, adding in your Swiss chard, garlic and spinach. Cook for five minutes, and then remove it from heat. Set it to the side.
3. Whisk your celery, eggs, sea salt and red pepper flakes. Add this to your pan.
4. Make sure you spread the egg evenly, cooking for about two minutes.
5. Add your greens over your egg before serving.

Nutrition Facts:
Calories: 227
Fat: 20.7 Grams
Net Carbs: 2.9 Grams
Protein: 9.3 Grams

Simple Breakfast Bake

Serves: 8

Time: 1 Hour

Ingredients:
- 8 Eggs
- 1 lb. Homemade Sausage
- 1 Tablespoon Olive Oil + Extra
- 2 Cups Spaghetti Squash, Cooked
- 1 Tablespoon Oregano, Fresh & Chopped
- ½ Cup Cheddar Cheese, Shredded
- Sea Salt & Black Pepper to Taste

Directions:
1. Start by heating your oven to 375, and then grease a 9x13 pan with your oil. Set your dish to the side, and then take out an ovenproof skillet.
2. Heat your skillet over medium-high heat with your olive oil.
3. Brown your sausage, cooking all the way through. This should take roughly five minutes.
4. Whisk your eggs, oregano, and squash together. Season with sea salt and black pepper before placing this mixture to the side.
5. Add your cooked sausage to your egg mixture, stirring to combine.
6. Pour this mix into your pan.
7. Sprinkle the cheese on top, and cover loosely with aluminum foil.
8. Bake for thirty minutes, and then remove your foil. Bake for another fifteen minutes.
9. Allow it to cool for ten minutes before serving.

Nutrition Facts:

Calories: 303

Fat: 24 Grams

Net Carbs: 3 Grams

Protein: 17 Grams

Green Smoothie Bowl

Serves: 1
Time: 5 Minutes
Ingredients:

- 1 Cup Spinach, Chopped
- 1 Tablespoon Greek Yogurt, Plain
- 2 Tablespoons Coconut Oil
- ¼ Cup Almond Milk, Unsweetened
- ¼ Teaspoon Stevia Powder

Directions:

1. Place all ingredients into a blender, blending until smooth.

Nutrition Facts:

Calories: 394
Fat: 42 Grams
Net Carbs: 3.2 Grams
Protein: 4.2 Grams

Poached Eggs & Spinach

Serves: 2

Time: 25 Minutes

Ingredients:

- 2 Eggs
- 1 lb. Spinach, Chopped Fine
- ¼ Teaspoon Garlic Powder
- 4 Tablespoons Olive Oil
- ¼ Teaspoon Rosemary, Dried
- ½ Teaspoon Sea Salt, Fine

Directions:

1. Heat your oil in a skillet over medium-high heat. Add in your spinach, seasoning with garlic. Fry for three to four minutes, and then crack your eggs into the pan. Season your eggs with sea salt and rosemary, frying for four minutes.
2. Flip or scramble, cooking for three more minutes.
3. Serve warm.

Nutrition Facts:

Calories: 297

Fat: 26.9 Grams

Net Carbs: 3.8 Grams

Protein: 12.1 Grams

Pancakes & Raspberry Cream

Serves: 4
Time: 15 Minutes
Ingredients:
Pancakes:

- ¼ Cup Coconut Oil, Softened
- 3 Tablespoons Almond Flour
- 3 Tablespoons Greek Yogurt, Plain
- 4 Eggs
- 1 Teaspoon Vanilla Extract, Pure
- 1 Teaspoon Baking Powder
- ¼ Cup Water
- 1 Tablespoon Stevia Powder

Cream:

- 1 Cup Greek Yogurt
- 2 Tablespoons Whipped Cream
- 3 Tablespoons Skim Milk
- 2 Teaspoons Raspberry Extract, Sugar Free
- ½ Teaspoon Stevia Powder

Directions:

1. Start by mixing all pancake ingredients in a blender, pulsing until smooth.
2. Heat your griddle, and then spray with cooking spray.
3. Add ¼ cup of your batter, cooking for two minutes. Repeat to use up all of your batter.
4. To make your raspberry cream, combine all ingredients in a blender, blending until smooth. This makes four servings.

Nutrition Facts (Pancakes):
Calories: 200
Fat: 19 Grams
Net Carbs: 1.5 Grams
Protein: 6.9 Grams

Nutrition Facts (Raspberry Cream):
Calories: 64

Fat: 3.3 Grams
Net Carbs: 2.8 Grams
Protein: 5.6 Grams

Eggs Baked in Avocado

Serves: 2
Time: 25 Minutes
Ingredients:

- 1 Avocado, Halved & Pitted
- 2 Eggs
- ½ Teaspoon Rosemary, Dried
- 1 Teaspoon Thyme, Dried
- 2 Tablespoons Olive Oil
- ½ Teaspoon Celery, Dried
- ¼ Teaspoon Red Pepper Flakes
- 1 Teaspoon Sea Salt, Fine

Directions:

1. Start by turning your oven to 400, and then line a baking sheet with parchment paper.
2. Cut your avocado in half removing the pit and brushing it down with your oil.
3. Pour your eggs into each hole, sprinkling with your seasoning.
4. Bake for fifteen minutes. Your eggs should be set, and serve warm.

Nutrition Facts:
Calories: 391
Fat: 38.1 Grams
Net Carbs: 2.5 Grams
Protein: 7.5 Grams

Shrimp & Eggs

Serves: 2
Time: 25 Minutes
Ingredients:

- 2 Ounces Cream Cheese
- 4 Eggs
- 7 Ounces Shrimp, Cleaned
- 2 Tablespoons Butter
- 2 Tablespoons Cilantro, Fresh & Chopped Fine
- 1 Teaspoon Basil, Fresh & Chopped
- ¼ Teaspoon Sea Salt, Fine

Directions:

1. Start by melting your butter in as skillet, adding your onion and sprinkling with sea salt. Fry for one minute, and then add in your shrimp. Cook for about eight minutes.
2. Crack your eggs in a bowl, and then add in your cilantro, basil, cream cheese and sea salt. Whisk together before adding it into your pan.
3. Cook for two more minutes, and serve warm.

Nutrition Facts:
Calories: 449
Fat: 31.9 Grams
Net Carbs: 3.5 Grams
Protein: 36.2 Grams

Keto Waffles

Serves: 5
Time: 25 Minutes
Ingredients:
- 1 Teaspoon Vanilla Extract, Pure
- 1 Tablespoon Olive Oil
- 1 Tablespoon Whipped Cream
- 1 Cup Cream Cheese
- 2 Tablespoons Butter, Softened
- 1 Tablespoon Almond Flour
- 4 Eggs, Separated
- 1 Egg White
- 2 Tablespoons Oat Bran

Directions:
1. Start by mixing your cream cheese, egg whites, and butter in a bowl. Mix for two minutes on high speed.
2. Add in your yolks, doing so one at a time, and continuing to beat as you do.
3. Add in your oat, bran, flour, vanilla extract and whipped cream, continuing to beat.
4. Grease a waffle iron, and then pour ¼ cup of the batter in. cook for two minutes, and continue until you're done with your batter.
5. Serve with more whipped cream while still warm.

Nutrition Facts:
Calories: 313
Fat: 28.9 Grams
Net Carbs: 3.9 Grams
Protein: 9.7 Grams

Mushroom Frittata

Serves: 6
Time: 25 Minutes
Ingredients:

- 2 Tablespoons Olive Oil
- 1 cup Mushrooms, Fresh & Sliced
- 1 Cup Spinach, Fresh & Shredded
- 6 Bacon Slices, Cooked & Chopped
- 10 Eggs, Beaten
- ½ Cup Goat Cheese, Crumbled
- Sea Salt & Black Pepper to Taste

Directions:

1. Start by heating your oven to 350.
2. Take an ovenproof skillet, heating it over medium-high heat and tossing in your olive oil.
3. Cook your mushrooms until lightly browned, which should take about three minutes.
4. Add in your bacon and spinach, cooking until your spinach wilts. This should take another minute.
5. Add in your eggs, cooking and lifting them up so that the egg flows underneath. This should take another three to four minutes.
6. Sprinkle your goat cheese on top, seasoning with sea salt and black pepper.
7. Bake in your oven until browned, which should take about fifteen minutes.
8. Let it cool for five minutes before slicing to serve.

Nutrition Facts:
Calories: 316
Fat: 27 Grams
Net Carbs: 1 Grams
Protein: 16 Grams

Cheesy Scrambled Eggs

Serves: 2
Time: 10 Minutes
Ingredients:
- 3 Tablespoons Butter
- 4 Eggs, Large
- ¼ Cup Cheddar Cheese, Grated
- 2 Tablespoons Dill, Fresh & Finely Chopped
- ¼ Teaspoon Sea Salt, Fine

Directions:
1. Start by melting your butter in a skillet, using medium-high heat.
2. In a bowl, whisk your eggs, cheddar cheese, sea salt and dill together.
3. Pour the mixture into your heated skillet, scrambling until done.
4. Serve warm.

Nutrition Fact:
Calories: 361
Fat: 32 Grams
Net Carbs: 2.3 Grams
Protein: 16.9 Grams

Cashew & Lemon Smoothie

Serves: 1
Time: 5 Minutes
Ingredients:
- 1 Cup Cashew Milk, Unsweetened
- ¼ Cup Lemon Juice, Fresh
- ¼ Cup Heavy Whipping Cream
- 1 Scoop Protein Powder, Plain
- 1 Teaspoon Sweetener
- 1 Tablespoon Coconut Oil

Directions:
1. Blend all ingredients until smooth before serving.

Nutrition Facts:
Calories: 503
Fat: 45 Grams
Net Carbs: 11 Grams
Protein: 29 Grams

Artichoke & Bacon Omelet

Serves: 4
Time: 20 Minutes
Ingredients:

- ½ Cup Artichoke Hearts, Chopped
- ¼ Cup Onion, Chopped
- 1 Tablespoon Olive Oil
- 2 Tablespoons Heavy Whipping Cream
- 6 Eggs, Beaten
- 8 Bacon Slices, Cooked & Chopped
- Sea Salt & Black Pepper to Taste

Directions:

1. Start by whisking your eggs, heavy cream, and bacon together before setting it to the side.
2. Place a skillet over medium-high heat, heating up your olive oil.
3. Cook your onion until its tender, which will take about three minutes.
4. Add your egg mix into the skillet, swirling to cook for a full minute.
5. Lift your egg so that the uncooked egg flows underneath, cooking for another two minutes.
6. Add your artichoke hearts on top before flipping your omelet, cooking for another four minutes. Your egg should be firm, and then flip it again so that your artichoke hearts are on top.
7. Take your omelet out of the skillet, and then quarter it. Season with salt and pepper before serving.

Nutrition Facts:
Calories: 435
Fat: 39 Grams
Net Carbs: 3 Grams
Protein: 17 Grams

Breakfast Burrito

Serves: 3
Time: 20 Minutes
Ingredients:
- 2 Tablespoons Olive Oil
- 2 Cloves Garlic, Minced
- ½ Cup Zucchini, Chopped
- 1/3 Cup Button Mushrooms, Sliced
- 2 Eggs
- 1/8 Teaspoon Chili Pepper
- ¼ Teaspoon Cayenne Pepper
- 2 Tablespoons Salsa, Sugar Free
- 3 Tortilla Shells, Low Carb

Directions:
1. Start by adding your oil to a skillet over medium-high heat. Add in your zucchini, frying for four to five minutes.
2. Add in your chili pepper, cayenne, and garlic, stirring before cooking for two more minutes. You'll need to stir constantly to keep it from burning.
3. Crack your eggs into your skillet, scrambling until done.
4. Divide between tortillas, drizzling with salsa and serving warm.

Nutrition Facts:
Calories: 166
Fat: 13.2 Grams
Net Carbs: 3.7 Grams
Protein: 6 Grams

Easy Salmon Spread

Serves: 4
Time: 15 Minutes
Ingredients:

- 4 Ounces Smoked Salmon, Minced
- 2 Tablespoons Sesame Oil
- ¼ Cup Cream
- 1 Tablespoon Sour Cream
- 1 Tablespoon Lemon Juice, Fresh
- ¼ Cup Parsley, Fresh & Chopped
- ½ Teaspoon Sea Salt, Fine
- 2 Cloves Garlic, Minced

Directions:

1. Start by combining your sour cream and cream cheese. Whisk together before adding in your oil, lemon juice, garlic, smoked salmon, sea salt and parsley. Beat for two minutes.
2. Serve chilled.

Nutrition Facts:

Calories: 310
Fat: 27.6 Grams
Net Carbs: 2.4 Grams
Protein: 13.2 Grams

Crusted Goat Cheese

Serves: 4
Time: 15 Minutes
Ingredients:
- 6 Ounces Walnuts, Chopped
- 1 Teaspoon Thyme, Fresh & Chopped
- 1 Tablespoon Parsley, Fresh & Chopped
- 1 Tablespoon Oregano, Fresh & Chopped
- ¼ Teaspoon Black Pepper
- 8 Ounces Goat Cheese

Directions:
1. Start by adding your thyme, parsley, oregano, walnuts and pepper in a food processor. Pulse until chopped fine.
2. Pour your mixture onto a plate, rolling your goat cheese log in it.
3. Wrap your cheese in plastic, storing it until you're ready to slice and serve.

Nutrition Facts:
Calories: 304
Fat: 28 Grams
Net Carbs: 2 Grams
Protein: 12 Grams

Shrimp & Collar Greens

Serves: 5
Time: 1 Hour 30 Minutes
Ingredients:
- 2 lbs. Collard Greens, Chopped
- 7 Ounces Octopus
- 1 lb. Shrimp, Whole
- 1 Tomato, Peeled & Chopped Fine
- 3 Cups Fish Stock
- 1 Tablespoon Butter
- 3 Tablespoons Olive Oil
- 3 Cloves Garlic, Minced
- ½ Teaspoon Thyme, dried
- 2 Tablespoons Parsley, Fresh & Chopped Fine
- 1 Teaspoon Sea Salt, Fine

Directions:
1. Put your place octopus in a pressure cooker, adding water to cover it. Cook for forty-five minutes, and then use a quick release.
2. Allow it to cool before chopping.
3. Rinse your shrimp, placing them in a deep pot. Add your tomato, fish stock and chopped octopus. Bring it to a boil, cooking for five to seven minutes.
4. Take it off heat, and then drain it before setting it aside.
5. Grease a skillet with your oil and then add in your garlic, stir frying for a minute.
6. Add in your collard greens, cooking for five minutes. You'll need to stir constantly to keep it from burning.
7. Add in your shrimp, butter, octopus, sea salt and parsley.
8. Cook for another three minutes, stirring often.
9. Serve warm.

Nutrition Facts:
Calories: 308
Fat: 17.5 Grams
Net Carbs: 7 Grams
Protein: 28.3 Grams

Parmesan Crackers

Serves: 1
Time: 15 Minutes
Ingredients:
- 1 Teaspoon Butter
- 8 Ounces Parmesan Cheese, Grated Fresh

Directions:
1. Start by heating your oven to 400.
2. Take out a baking sheet, lining it with parchment paper and lightly greasing that paper with your butter.
3. Spoon the parmesan into eight mounds on the baking sheet.
4. Bake until the edges are browned, which will take about five minutes.
5. Remove from baking sheet, and allow it to cool.

Nutrition Facts (1 Cracker):
Calories: 133
Fat: 1 Grams
Net Carbs: 1 Gram
Protein: 11 Grams

Easy Meatballs

Serves: 4
Time: 25 Minutes
Ingredients:
- 1 lb. Ground Beef, Lean
- 1 Teaspoon Sea Salt, Fine
- ½ Teaspoon Ground Black Pepper
- 1 Onion, Finely Chopped
- 2 Eggs
- ½ Teaspoon Cumin
- ¼ Cup Almond Milk
- 3 Tablespoons Olive Oil
- 1 Tablespoon Coriander, Fresh
- 2 Tablespoons Buckwheat Groats

Directions:
1. Start by placing two slices of keto bread in a bowl, adding ¼ cup of water. Let it stand for five minutes.
2. Combine your ground beef, milk, and coriander, a tablespoon of oil, cumin, buckwheat groats, sea salt, pepper and eggs together.
3. Add in your soaked bread, and then shape into balls with ¼ cup of the mixture.
4. Flatten each in the palm of your hand, and then heat up your remaining oil in a skillet.
5. Add in your meatballs, frying for three to four minutes.
6. Serve warm.

Nutrition Facts:
Calories: 379
Fat: 23.4 Grams
Net Carbs: 2.9 Grams
Protein: 37.9 Grams

Cheesy Deviled Eggs

Serves: 12
Time: 20 Minutes
Ingredients:

- 6 Eggs, Hardboiled & Peeled
- ¼ Cup Creamy Mayonnaise, Keto Friendly
- ½ Teaspoon Dijon Mustard
- ¼ Cup Swiss Cheese, Shredded Fine
- ¼ Avocado, Chopped
- 6 Bacon Slices, Cooked & Chopped
- Black Pepper to Taste

Directions:

1. Start by halving your eggs lengthwise.
2. Remove the yolks, placing them in a bowl. Put your hollowed whites on a plate.
3. Mash your yolks, adding in all other ingredients but your egg whites and bacon. Mix well.
4. Spoon the mixture into each egg white, topping with chopped bacon.
5. Serve chilled.

Nutrition Facts:

Calories: 85
Fat: 7 Grams
Net Carbs: 2 Grams
Protein: 6 Grams

Tuna Salad

Serves: 2
Time: 30 Minutes
Ingredients:

- 1 Cup Tuna, Canned & Oil Free
- 3 Eggs, Boiled
- 1 Cup Baby Spinach, Chopped Fine
- ½ Cup Goat Cheese, Fresh
- ½ Carrot, Sliced
- 1 Tablespoon Lemon Juice, Fresh
- ½ Teaspoon Sea Salt, Fine

Directions:

1. Start by putting your eggs in boiling water, cooking for twelve minutes. Remove from heat, draining.
2. Allow them to chill to room temperature, and then peel them.
3. Chop your eggs, and then add all remaining ingredients together.

Nutrition Facts:
Calories: 297
Fat: 16 Grams
Net Carbs: 2.2 Grams
Protein: 34.1 Grams

Crab Stuffed Avocado

Serves: 2
Time: 20 Minutes
Ingredients:
- 1 Avocado, Peeled, Pitted & Halved Lengthwise
- ½ Teaspoon Lemon Juice, Fresh
- 4 ½ Ounces Dungeness Crab meat
- ½ Cup Cream Cheese
- ¼ Cup Cucumber, Peeled & Chopped
- ¼ Cup Red Bell Pepper, Chopped
- ½ Scallion, Chopped
- 1 Teaspoon Cilantro, Fresh & Chopped
- Sea Salt & Black Pepper to Taste

Directions:
1. Place your lemon juice over the avocado edges, and then place your avocado on a plate.
2. In a bowl, stir together your cream cheese, red pepper, crab meat, scallion, cucumber, sea salt, black pepper and cilantro. Mix until well combined.
3. Divide your mixture between your avocados, and chill to serve.

Nutrition Facts:
Calories: 389
Fat: 31 Grams
Net Carbs: 5 Grams
Protein: 19 Grams

Veal Skewers

Serves: 4

Time: 30 Minutes

Ingredients:

- 1 lb. Veal, Ground
- 2 Tablespoons Almond Flour
- 3 Eggs
- 2 Cloves Garlic, Crushed
- ½ Tablespoon Cumin Seeds
- 1 Tablespoon Coriander Seeds
- 1 Tablespoon Olive Oil
- 1 Teaspoon Mint, Dried
- 1 Teaspoon Sea Salt, Fine
- ½ Teaspoon Ground Black Pepper
- ¼ Tablespoon Cayenne Pepper

Directions:

1. Soak your wooden skewers for fifteen to twenty minutes.
2. Take a skillet, placing it over medium-high heat.
3. Mix your lamb, eggs, garlic, almond flour, coriander seeds, oil, mint, cumin seeds, cayenne, and sea salt and pepper together.
4. Mix well, shaping into balls that are about two inches in diameter.
5. Arrange your balls on your skewers, browning for three to four minutes on each side.

Nutrition Facts:

Calories: 377

Fat: 24 Grams

Net Carbs: 5 Grams

Protein: 33.7 Grams

Fish Curry

Serves: 4

Time: 35 Minutes

Ingredients:

- 2 Tablespoons Coconut Oil
- 2 Teaspoon Garlic, Minced
- 1 ½ Tablespoons Ginger, Fresh & Grated
- 1 Tablespoon Curry Powder
- 2 Cups Coconut Milk
- ½ Teaspoon Ground Cumin
- 16 Ounces White Fish, Firm & Cut into 1 Inch Chunks
- 1 Cup Kale, Shredded
- 2 Tablespoons Cilantro, Fresh & Chopped

Directions:

1. Start by placing a saucepan over medium heat, adding in your coconut oil.
2. Once it's hot, add in your garlic and ginger. Sauté for two minutes. It should brown.
3. Stir in the coconut milk, bringing it to a boil.
4. Reduce your heat to low, and simmer for five minutes before adding in your fish.
5. Cook for about ten minutes, and then stir in your cilantro and kale. Allow it to simmer and wilt, which will take about two minutes.
6. Serve warm.

Nutrition Facts:

Calories: 416

Fat: 31 Grams

Net Carbs: 4 Grams

Protein: 26 Grams

Braised Leeks & Beef

Serves: 4
Time: 1 Hour 20 Minutes
Ingredients:
- 1 Bay Leaf
- 1 lb. Beef Stew Meat
- 2 Leeks, Large
- 1 Carrot, Sliced
- 1 Onion, Sliced
- 1 Cup Celery Leaves, Chopped
- 1 Teaspoon Sea Salt, Fine
- ¼ Teaspoon Ground Black Pepper
- 2 Tablespoons Vegetable Oil
- 3 Tablespoon Olive Oil
- ½ Teaspoon Rosemary, Dried

Directions:
1. Start by greasing the bottom of your pressure cooker with your vegetable oil. Sprinkle your meat with salt, placing it inside. Add in your carrots, celery, bay leaf, and onions. Add enough water to cover, and then close the lid.
2. Steam for forty-five minutes, and then release the steam.
3. Separate your meat, setting it to the side.
4. Rinse your leeks, chopping it to bite sized pieces.
5. Heat up your olive oil using medium-high heat in a skillet. Add in your leeks, cooking for ten minutes.
6. Place it in a deep pot, adding all ingredients together. Stir until it comes to a boil, cooking for five more minutes. You'll need to stir constantly.

Nutrition Facts:
Calories: 389
Fat: 24.5 Grams
Net Carbs: 5.6 Grams
Protein: 35.1 Grams

Bacon & Chicken Burgers

Serves: 6
Time: 35 Minutes
Ingredients:

- 1 lb. Chicken, Ground
- 8 Bacon Slices, Chopped
- ¼ Cup Almonds, Ground
- ¼ Teaspoon Sea Salt, Fine
- 1 Teaspoon Basil, Fresh & Chopped
- Pinch Black Pepper
- 4 Lettuce Leaves, Large
- 2 Tablespoons Coconut Oil
- 1 Avocado, Peeled, Pitted & Sliced

Directions:

1. Start by heating your oven to 350, and then line a baking sheet using parchment paper.
2. In a bowl, combine your chicken, bacon, basil, sea salt, black pepper and ground almonds. Make sure to mix well, and then form the mixture into six patties.
3. Place a skillet with your coconut oil over medium-high heat.
4. Sear your patties for about three minutes on each side.
5. Put your patties on your baking sheet, baking for fifteen minutes.
6. Serve on lettuce leaves topped with your avocado slices.

Nutrition Facts:
Calories: 374
Fat: 33 Grams
Net Carbs: 1 Grams
Protein: 18 Grams

Grilled Mackerel & Spinach

Serves: 4

Time: 40 Minutes

Ingredients:

- 4 Mackerels, Skin On
- 1 lb. Spinach, Fresh & Torn
- ¼ Cup Olive Oil, Divided in Half
- 3 Cloves Garlic, Crushed
- 1 Teaspoon Rosemary, Dried
- 1 Lemon, Juiced
- 1 Teaspoon Sea Salt, Fine
- 2 Sprigs Mint Leaves, Chopped

Directions:

1. Start by heating up a grill pan over medium-high heat. Brush it down with your oil.
2. In a bowl, combine half of your oil with your mint, garlic, and rosemary and lemon juice. Brush your fixture over with this mixture, and then grill for five minutes per side.
3. Heat up the remaining oil over medium-high heat in a skillet, adding your spinach. Sprinkle with sea salt, stir frying for five to seven minutes.
4. Serve your fish and spinach together while warm.

Nutrition Facts:

Calories: 372

Fat: 28.8 Grams

Net Carbs: 3.2 Grams

Protein: 24.5 Grams

Lettuce Wraps with Salmon

Serves: 4
Time: 30 Minutes
Ingredients:

- 1 lb. Salmon
- 3 Eggs, Boiled
- ¼ Cup Fire Roasted Tomatoes, Diced
- 1 Teaspoon Italian Seasoning
- 2 Tablespoon Red Onion, Chopped Fine
- ¼ Teaspoon Red Pepper Flakes
- ½ Teaspoon Sea Salt, Fine
- 3 Tablespoons Olive Oil
- 8 Lettuce Leaves, Large
- ½ Cup Chicken Stock

Directions:

1. Start by heating up your oil in a pan over medium-high heat.
2. Add in your fillet, browning for three minutes on each side.
3. Stir in your sea salt, Italian seasoning, tomatoes and red pepper flakes.
4. Pour your fish stock in, bringing it to ab oil.
5. Cook until the liquid evaporates, and then remove from heat.
6. Chop with a knife, and then prepare your lettuce leaves.
7. Divide your salmon between each, and wrap before serving.

Nutrition Facts:
Calories: 302
Fat: 21.7 Grams
Net Carbs: 1.1 Grams
Protein: 27 Grams

Beef Skewers

Serves: 4

Time: 25 Minutes

Ingredients:

- 1 lb. Beef Sirloin Tips, Cubed into 2 Inch Pieces
- 3 Tablespoons Worcestershire Sauce
- ½ Cup Olive Oil
- 2 Tablespoons Lemon Juice, Fresh
- 1 Tablespoon Dijon Mustard
- ½ Teaspoon Stevia
- ¼ Ground Black Pepper
- 1 Teaspoon Garlic Powder

Directions:

1. Start by combining your Worcestershire sauce, oil, lemon juice, garlic powder, Dijon mustard, black pepper and stevia together.
2. Put your beef in a Ziploc bag, and then pour in your garlic mixture.
3. Seal, and then allow your steak to marinate for twenty to forty-five minutes.
4. Divide your beef between skewers, and then preheat a grill pan over high heat.
5. Put your skewers on it, and then cook for three minutes per side.
6. Serve warm.

Nutrition Facts:

Calories: 445

Fat: 32.5 Grams

Net Carbs: 2.9 Grams

Protein: 34.8 Grams

Spicy Salmon Frittata

Serves: 2
Time: 30 Minutes
Ingredients:

- 1 Tablespoon Coconut Oil
- 1 Red Onion, Chopped
- 1 Green Pepper, Chopped
- 2 Cloves Garlic, Minced
- 1 ½ Cups Cherry Tomatoes
- ½ Teaspoon Paprika
- ½ Cup Salmon
- 1 Teaspoon Cumin
- 6 Eggs, Beaten
- Sea Salt & Black Pepper to Taste
- 2 Tablespoons Cilantro, Fresh & Chopped

Directions:

1. Start by heating your oven to 350, and then melt your butter in a skillet that's oven safe.
2. Sauté your red onion and green pepper, stirring in your garlic. Cook for two minutes, and then add in your sea salt, pepper, cumin and paprika. Cook for another minute.
3. Stir in your tomatoes, cooking until they soften.
4. Add in your salmon, and then add your eggs over it.
5. Season with sea salt and black pepper, baking for fifteen minutes.
6. Serve garnished with your fresh cilantro.

Nutrition Facts:
Calories: 344
Fat: 22 Grams
Net Carbs: 12.2 Grams
Protein: 23.5 Grams

Catfish with Rosemary

Serves: 2

Time: 50 Minutes

Ingredients:
- 1 lb. Catfish Fillet
- 12 Cup Parsley, Fresh & Chopped Fine
- 2 Tablespoons Lemon Juice, Fresh
- 2 Cloves Garlic, Crushed
- 1 Onion, Chopped Fine
- 1 Tablespoon Dill, Chopped Fine
- 1 Tablespoon Rosemary, Fresh & Chopped
- ¼ Cup Apple Cider Vinegar
- 2 Tablespoons Dijon Mustard
- 1 Cup Olive Oil

Directions:
1. Start by combining your lemon juice, garlic, onion, parsley, rosemary, apple cider vinegar, dill and olive oil. Stir well.
2. Submerge your fillet in the mixture, letting it marinate for thirty minutes.
3. Heat a skillet over medium-high heat. Remove your fillets from the fridge, reserving the marinade.
4. Grill your fish for four minutes on each side. You'll use the grilled marinade to keep them from burning.
5. Serve warm.

Nutrition Fact:

Calories: 413

Fat: 24.9 Grams

Net Carbs: 6.6 Grams

Protein: 37.1 Grams

Citrus Tuna

Serves: 4

Time: 1 Hour 10 Minutes

Ingredients:

- ¼ Cup Coriander Leaves, Fresh & Chopped
- 4 Tuna Steaks, About a Pound
- 3 Cloves Garlic, Minced
- ½ Cup Olive Oil
- 2 Tablespoons Lemon Juice, Fresh
- ½ Teaspoon Cumin, Ground
- ½ Teaspoon Smoked Paprika
- ½ Teaspoon Chili Powder
- Sea Salt & Black Pepper to Taste

Directions:

1. Start by adding your coriander, paprika, cumin, chili powder, garlic, and lemon juice together in a food processor. Pulse until well combined, and then gradually add in your oil, mixing until smooth.
2. Place the mixture in a bowl, and then toss your fish in. make sure it's coated evenly, and allow it to marinate in the fridge for at least an hour.
3. Remove your fish, and then lightly brush your grill down with oil.
4. Grill for three to four minutes per side.
5. Serve warm.

Nutrition Facts:

Calories: 433

Fat: 32.6 Grams

Net Carbs: 1 Gram

Protein: 34.3 Grams

Chicken Thighs & Mushrooms

Serves: 2

Time: 30 Minutes

Ingredients:
- 2 Chicken Thighs, 7 Ounces Each & Skin On
- 7 Ounces Button Mushrooms
- 1 Teaspoon Rosemary, Fresh & Chopped Fine
- 2 Cloves Garlic, Crushed
- 3 Tablespoons Olive Oil
- ½ Teaspoon Sea Salt, Fine
- 1 Tablespoon Butter
- 1 Tablespoon Italian Seasoning

Directions:
1. Rub your meat down with your sea salt, and then grease a skillet with a tablespoon of your oil.
2. Add your rosemary, mushrooms, and Italian seasoning to your pan. Cook for five minutes over medium heat, and then stir in your butter. Remove it from heat, setting it to the side.
3. Turn your oven to 350, and then line a baking sheet with parchment paper.
4. Brush your chicken thighs with oil, baking for thirty-five minutes.
5. Remove your thighs from the oven at thirty minutes, and then coat with your mushroom mixture. Bake for another five to seven minutes.

Nutrition Facts:

Calories: 471

Fat: 27 Grams

Net Carbs: 3.3 Grams

Protein: 52.5 Grams

Easy Lobster

Serves: 2

Time: 40 Minutes

Ingredients:

- ¼ Teaspoon Red Pepper Flakes
- Sea Salt & Black Pepper to Taste
- ¼ Cup Lemon Juice, Fresh
- ¼ Cup Olive Oil
- 1 lb. Lobster Tails

Directions:

1. Start by heating your oven to 350, and then line a baking sheet with parchment paper.
2. Rinse your lobster tails, patting them dry. Put your lobster tails onto the baking sheet.
3. Combine your red pepper flakes, sea salt, black pepper, oil and lemon juice together, brushing the mixture over your lobster tails.
4. Bake for ten minutes, and then remove your baking sheet for the oven.
5. Flip your lobster tails over, and then brush down with the remaining mixture before baking for another fifteen minutes.

Nutrition Facts:

Calories: 428

Fat: 27.4 Grams

Net Carbs: 0.3 Grams

Protein: 43.4 Grams

Braised Short Ribs

Serves: 4

Time: 2 Hours 30 Minutes

Ingredients:

- 4 Beef Short Ribs, 4 Ounces Each
- Sea Salt & Black Pepper to Taste
- 1 Tablespoon Olive Oil
- ½ Cup Red Wine, Dry
- 2 Teaspoons Garlic, Minced
- 3 Cups Beef Stock

Directions:

1. Start by heating your oven to 325, and then season your ribs with sea salt and black pepper.
2. Put them in an ovenproof skillet over medium-high heat. Add in your olive oil.
3. Sear your ribs until they're browned on all sides, which should take about six minutes.
4. Transfer your ribs to a plate.
5. Place your garlic in the skillet, cooking for about three minutes.
6. Whisk your red wine in, deglazing the pan.
7. Simmer your wine for two minutes, which should reduce it slightly.
8. Add in your ribs, beef stock, and any juices that are on the plate back into your skillet. Bring your mixture to a boil, and then place it in the oven. Cook for two hours.
9. Serve your ribs with a spoonful of liquid over them.

Nutrition Facts:

Calories: 481

Fat: 38 Grams

Net Carbs: 2 Grams

Protein: 29 Grams

Veal Salad

Serves: 4
Time: 25 Minutes
Ingredients:

- 1 Tomato, Large
- 2 Veal Cutlets, Boneless & Chopped
- ½ Cup Cabbage, Grated
- 1 Green Pepper
- 2 Tablespoons Olive Oil
- Sea Salt to Taste

Directions:

1. Start by heating up your olive oil over medium heat. Fry your cutlets for ten minutes per side.
2. Remove from heat, and then rinse your vegetables and drain them.
3. Transfer to a bowl, topping with meat.
4. Season with oil and sea salt.

Nutrition Facts:

Calories: 200
Fat: 13.1 Grams
Net Carbs: 2.8 Grams
Protein: 16.6 Grams

Beef Liver with Red Peppers

Serves: 4
Time: 20 Minutes
Ingredients:
- 2 Cloves Garlic, Crushed
- 1 lb. Beef Liver, Sliced Thin
- 3 Tablespoons Olive Oil
- 1 Tablespoon Mint, Fresh & Chopped Fine
- 1 Teaspoon Sea Salt, Fine
- ½ Tablespoon Cayenne Pepper
- ½ Teaspoon Italian Seasoning

Directions:
1. Start by heating a grill pan over medium-high heat.
2. Rinse your liver using cold water, and then pat it dry with a paper towel.
3. Use a sharp knife to remove any tough veins, and then slice your liver.
4. In a bowl combine your garlic, olive oil, cayenne, Italian seasoning, mint and sea salt. Mix well, and then brush over your liver.
5. Cook your liver for three to four minutes per side.

Nutrition Facts:
Calories: 295
Fat: 16.1 Grams
Net Carbs: 6.6 Grams
Protein: 30.3 Grams

Basil & Tomato Stew

Serves: 8

Time: 1 Hour 15 Minutes

Ingredients:

- 1 Cup Fire Roasted Tomatoes, Diced
- 2 lbs. Mixed Fish, Salmon, Whiting Fish & Mackerel
- 1 Tablespoon Basil, Dried
- 6 Cups Fish Stock
- 6 Stalks Celery, Chopped
- 6 Tablespoons Tomato Paste
- 3 Carrots, Sliced
- 3 Tablespoons Olive Oil
- 1 Onion, Chopped Fine
- 6 Cloves Garlic, Minced

Directions:

1. Heat your olive oil in a skillet over medium high heat. Add in your onion, cooking until translucent. Add in your garlic, tomato paste, celery, carrots and basil. Stir, cooking for two minutes.
2. Add in your fire roasted tomatoes and a cup of your fish stock. Bring it to a boil before removing the mixture from heat.
3. Transfer you mixture to a heavy bottomed pot, and then add in your fish as well as your remaining stock.
4. Cover, cooking over medium heat for forty-five minutes.

Nutrition Facts:

Calories: 324

Fat: 16.4 Grams

Net Carbs: 5.7 grams

Protein: 35.4 Grams

Cheeseburger Casserole

Serves: 6

Time: 50 Minutes

Ingredients:

- ½ Cup Heavy Whipping Cream
- 1 lb. Ground Beef, Lean
- ½ Cup Sweet Onion, Chopped
- 1 ½ Cups Aged Cheddar, Shredded & Divided
- 2 Teaspoons Garlic, Minced
- 1 Tomato, Large & Chopped
- 1 Teaspoon Basil, Fresh & Minced
- Sea Salt & Black Pepper to Taste

Directions:

1. Start by heating your oven to 350, and then put a large skillet over medium-high heat. Add in your ground beef, browning for six minutes. Drain any excess fat.
2. Add in your garlic and onion, cooking until tender. This should take about four minutes.
3. Place the mixture in a greased eight by eight pan.
4. Stir a cup of your shredded cheese, tomato, heavy cream, sea salt, black pepper and basil together. Make sure it's combined well.
5. Pour this mixture over your beef, and then top with your remaining cheese.
6. Bake for thirty minutes, and serve warm.

Nutrition Facts:

Calories: 410

Fat: 33 Grams

Net Carbs: 3 Grams

Protein: 20 Grams

Chicken Fillets

Serves: 4
Time: 30 Minutes
Ingredients:

- 1 lb. Chicken Breast, Boneless & Skinless
- ¼ Cup Apple Cider Vinegar
- ¼ Cup Olive Oil
- 1 Tablespoon Rosemary, Fresh & Chopped Fine
- 1 Teaspoon Oregano, Dried
- ½ Teaspoon Sea Salt, Fine
- 1 Teaspoon Cayenne Pepper

Directions:

1. Start by heating your grill to medium-high heat.
2. Rinse your meat and pat it dry. Slice into half inch slices, and set your chicken to the side.
3. Combine your apple cider, olive oil, cayenne, salt, oregano and rosemary together.
4. Brush your fillets with the mixture, grilling for seven minutes per side.
5. Serve warm.

Nutrition Facts:

Calories: 246
Fat: 15.7 Grams
Net Carbs: 0.6 Grams
Protein: 24.2 Grams

Peppered Beef

Serves: 4

Time: 2 Hours 5 Minutes

Ingredients:
- 1 lb. Beef Fillets, Chopped
- 3 Tablespoons Tomato Paste, Sugar Free
- 1 Onion, Peeled & Chopped Fine
- 1 Tablespoon Butter, Softened
- 2 Tablespoons Olive Oil
- 2 Tablespoons Parsley, Fresh & Chopped Fine
- Sea Salt & Black Pepper to Taste

Directions:
1. Start by greasing a pot with your olive oil. Add in your onions, cooking over medium-high heat. Cook for two to three minutes.
2. Add your meat, browning it for about five minutes.
3. Stir in your tomato paste, butter, sea salt, black pepper and parsley.
4. Add in enough water to cover it before reducing your heat to low.
5. Cook for one and a half hours, stirring on occasion.

Nutrition Facts:

Calories: 318

Fat: 17.1 Grams

Net Carbs: 3.9 Grams

Protein: 35.3 Grams

Beef Salad

Serves: 5
Time: 25 Minutes
Ingredients:

- 1 Tomato, Large & Sliced
- 1 lb. Rib Eye Steak, Boneless
- 7 Ounces Arugula, Fresh
- ¼ Cup Goat's Cheese, Fresh
- 5 Walnuts, Chopped
- 5 Hazelnuts, Chopped
- 5 Almonds, Chopped
- 3 Tablespoons Olive Oil
- 2 Tablespoons Red Wine Vinegar
- 1 Tablespoon Italian Seasoning

Directions:

1. Start by heating a grill to medium-high, and then brush your steak down with olive oil. Grill on one side for five to seven minutes. Flip, and then grill on the other side for four to five minutes.
2. Remove it from heat, allowing it to cool before slicing.
3. Whisk your Italian seasoning, red wine vinegar and olive oil together. Set this mixture to the side.
4. In a bowl, combine your arugula, goat's cheese, almonds, sliced tomato, walnuts, and hazelnuts together.
5. Top with your steak, and drizzle with your red wine mixture before serving.

Nutrition Facts:
Calories: 374
Fat: 28.7 Grams
Net Carbs: 2.2 Grams
Protein: 27.1 Grams

Mediterranean Shrimp

Serves: 4

Time: 15 Minutes

Ingredients:

- 1 Teaspoon Sea Salt, Fine
- 1 lb. Shrimp, Fresh & Whole
- 3 Cloves Garlic, Crushed
- 3 Tablespoons Olive Oil
- 3 Tablespoons Parsley, Fresh & Chopped Fine

Directions:

1. Start by rinsing and draining your shrimp. Pat it dry with a paper towel, and then heat up a grill pan over medium-high heat. Brush your grill pan with oil.
2. Add in your shrimp, and grill for three minutes per side.
3. Remove from heat, transferring your shrimp to a plate.
4. Top with garlic and parsley before seasoning with sea salt. Serve warm.

Nutrition Facts:

Calories: 186

Fat: 10.5 Grams

Net Carbs: 2.9 Grams

Protein: 21.5 Grams

Sea Bass with Lemon

Serves: 2
Time: 40 Minutes
Ingredients:
- 1 Tablespoon Olive Oil
- 2 Small Sea Bass, Cleaned & Gutted
- 4 Tablespoons Lemon Juice, Fresh
- 1 Tablespoon Rosemary, Dried
- 1 Teaspoon Sea Salt, Fine

Directions:
1. Start by heating your oven to 400. Prepare a baking sheet by lining it with parchment paper before placing it to the side.
2. Take a bowl, whisking your lemon juice, sea salt, rosemary and olive oil together.
3. Rinse your fish before patting it dry, and then rub the fish with your mixture.
4. Bake for twenty to twenty-five minutes.

Nutrition Facts:
Calories: 479
Fat: 32.9 Grams
Net Carbs: 0.1 Grams
Protein: 44.7 Grams

Stuffed Chicken Breasts

Serves: 2

Time: 55 Minutes

Ingredients:

- 1 lb. Chicken Breast, Boneless & Skinless
- ½ Cup Cottage Cheese
- 1 Cup Spinach, Fresh & Chopped
- 2 Tablespoon Sour Cream
- 1 Teaspoon Celery, Dried
- ½ Teaspoon Sea Salt, Fine
- ¼ Teaspoon Garlic Powder
- 1 Tablespoon Olive Oil

Directions:

1. Start by heating your oven to 400, lining a baking sheet with parchment paper before setting it to the side.
2. Take a skillet, greasing it with olive oil before placing it over medium-high heat.
3. Add in your garlic, spinach and salt. Stir, cooking it for two to three minutes.
4. Add in your sour cream and cottage cheese, cooking for a minute before removing it from heat.
5. Rinse your meat before patting it dry.
6. Make an incision into the chicken, and then stuff your chicken breast with the mixture.
7. Sprinkle with celery before baking for thirty-five minutes.

Nutrition Facts:

Calories: 400

Fat: 16.3 Grams

Net Carbs: 3 Grams

Protein: 56.7 Grams

Veal with Mushrooms

Serves: 4

Time: 50 Minutes

Ingredients:

- 1 lb. Button Mushrooms, Sliced Thin
- 1 lb. Veal Steaks
- 3 Tablespoons Olive Oil
- 1 Teaspoon Sea Salt, Fine
- ½ Teaspoon Black Pepper
- 1 Bay Leaf
- 1 Tablespoon Thyme, Dried

Directions:

1. Start by heating up your oil in a large skillet.
2. Add in your steaks, pouring a cup of water over it.
3. Bring it to a boil, and then add in your bay leaf. Reduce the heat to medium, and allow it to simmer for twenty-five minutes. Add more water if you need to.
4. Add in your button mushrooms once all of your water has evaporated.
5. Cook for ten minutes using medium heat, and serve warm.

Nutrition Facts:

Calories: 316

Fat: 18 Grams

Net Carbs: 2.9 Grams

Protein: 33.5 Grams

Easy Rosti

Serves: 8
Time: 30 Minutes
Ingredients:
- 8 Bacon Slices, Chopped
- 1 Cup Acorn Squash, Shredded
- 1 Cup Celeriac, Raw & Shredded
- 2 Tablespoons Parmesan Cheese, Grated
- 2 Teaspoons Garlic, Minced
- 1 Teaspoon Thyme, Fresh & Chopped
- 2 Tablespoons Butter
- Sea Salt & Black Pepper to Taste

Directions:
1. Start by heating a skillet over medium-high heat, cooking your bacon for about five minutes. It should become crispy.
2. In a bowl, mid your celeriac, squash, garlic, thyme and parmesan together. Season with sea salt and black pepper before setting the mixture to the side.
3. Remove your bacon, and mix it with your parmesan mixture.
4. Remove all but two tablespoons of fat from the skillet. Add in your butter, and reduce the heat to medium-low.
5. Transfer your mixture to the skillet, spreading it to form a round one inch patty.
6. Cook until the bottom is golden brown, which should take about five minutes.
7. Flip, and cook it for another five minutes.
8. Allow it to cool slightly before slicing to serve.

Nutrition Facts:
Calories: 171
Fat: 15 Grams
Net Carbs: 3 Grams
Protein: 5 Grams

Grilled Eel

Serves: 4

Time: 30 Minutes

Ingredients:

- 1 lb. Eel, Cleaned & Gutted
- 1 Tablespoon Thyme, Dried
- 1 Teaspoon Pink Himalayan Sea Salt
- 1 Cup Olive Oil
- 1 Tablespoon White Wine
- 1 Teaspoon Rosemary, Fresh & Chopped
- 1 Tablespoon Cilantro, Fresh & Chopped Fine

Directions:

1. Start by combining your olive oil, wine, rosemary, thyme, sea salt and cilantro. Stir well, and then brush your fish down with the mixture. Allow it to marinate in the fridge for an hour.
2. Drained from the marinade, and then lightly oil your grill. Turn it to high heat, and then place your eel on it, cooking for three to four minutes. It should become lightly charred.
3. Flip it over, and brush the marinade on the other side. Grill for five more minutes.
4. Serve warm.

Nutrition Facts:

Calories: 382

Fat: 29.7 Grams

Net Carbs: 0.3 Grams

Protein: 26.9 Grams

Portobello Pizza

Serves: 4
Time: 20 Minutes
Ingredients:

- ¼ Cup Olive Oil
- 4 Portobello Mushrooms, Stemmed Removed
- 1 Teaspoon Garlic, Minced
- 1 Tomato, Cut into 4 Slices
- 2 Teaspoon Basil, Fresh & Chopped
- 1 Cup Mozzarella Cheese, Shredded

Directions:

1. Start by heating your oven to broil, and then line a baking sheet with aluminum foil before setting it to the side.
2. In ab owl, toss your mushroom caps with your oil until they're coated. Make sure you don't break your mushrooms up.
3. Place the mushrooms on your baking sheet with the gill side down.
4. Broil until they're tender, which should take about two minutes.
5. Flip your mushrooms over, broiling for one more minute. Take your baking sheet out.
6. Top each mushroom with your tomato before sprinkling your basil and cheese over it.
7. Broil until your cheese is melted, which should take about a minute.
8. Serve warm.

Nutrition Facts:
Calories: 251
Fat: 20 Grams
Net Carbs: 4 Grams
Protein: 14 Grams

Bouillabaisse

Serves: 8

Time: 45 Minutes

Ingredients:

- 1 lb. Shrimp, Whole
- 1 lb. Red Mullet, Cleaned
- 1 lb. Tench Fillet
- 1 Mackerel, Cleaned
- 3 Tomatoes, Peeled & Chopped Rough
- 2 Onions, Chopped Fine
- 2 Stalks Celery, Sliced
- 2 Carrots, Grated
- 3 Tablespoons Olive Oil
- 4 Cups Fish Stock
- 1 Tablespoon Rosemary, Dried & Chopped Fine
- 1 Teaspoon Sea Salt, Fine

Directions:

1. Start by heating your oil in a saucepan, adding your celery, carrots and onion. Season with sea salt and rosemary, cooking for five minutes.
2. Add in your tomatoes, stirring well. Cook for seven minutes, stirring occasionally.
3. Add in your fish, scattering your shrimp over it, and then pour in your fish stock.
4. Bring the mixture to a boil before reducing your heat to medium-low. Cook for five to seven minutes.

Nutrition Facts:

Calories: 339

Fat: 14.4 Grams

Net Carbs: 6 Grams

Protein: 42.5 Grams

Glazed Trout

Serves: 5

Time: 35 Minutes

Ingredients:

- 2 lbs. Trout Fillets, Skin On
- 1 Tablespoon Lemon Juice, Fresh
- 2 Tablespoons Soy Sauce
- ½ Teaspoon Sea Salt, Fine
- 2 Teaspoons Dijon Mustard
- ½ Teaspoon Red Pepper Flakes

Directions:

1. Start by heating your oven to 425, and then line your baking sheet with parchment paper.
2. In a bowl, mix your lemon juice, soy sauce, red pepper flakes, sea salt and Dijon. Make sure it's well combined.
3. Rinse and dry your fillets, placing them on your baking sheet.
4. Spoon your mixture onto your fish, baking for fifteen to twenty minutes.
5. Serve warm.

Nutrition Facts:

Calories: 351

Fat: 15.5 Grams

Net Carbs: 0.6 Grams

Protein: 48.9 Grams

Garlic Green Beans

Serves: 4
Time: 20 Minutes
Ingredients:

- 1 lb. Green Beans, Trimmed
- 2 Tablespoons Olive Oil
- 1 Teaspoon Garlic, Minced
- ¼ Cup Parmesan Cheese, Grated Fine
- Sea Salt & Black Pepper to Taste

Directions:

1. Start by heating your oven to 425. Get out a baking sheet, lining it with aluminum foil.
2. In a bowl, toss your green beans with your garlic and olive oil. Make sure it's mixed well, and then season with sea salt and black pepper.
3. Spread your green beans on the baking sheet, roasting until they're tender. This should take ten minutes.
4. Top with parmesan cheese before serving.

Nutrition Facts:
Calories: 104
Fat: 9 Grams
Net Carbs: 1 Grams
Protein: 4 Grams

Cheesy Cauliflower Mash

Serves: 4

Time: 20 Minutes

Ingredients:

- 1 Head Cauliflower, Chopped
- ½ Cup Cheddar Cheese, Shredded
- 2 Tablespoon Butter, Room Temperature
- ¼ Cup Heavy Whipping Cream
- Sea Salt & Black Pepper to Taste

Directions:

1. Start by placing a large saucepan over high heat. Fill it three quarters full with water before bringing it to a boil.
2. Blanch your cauliflower, cooking until tender. It should take about five minutes, and then drain it.
3. Transfer your cauliflower to a food processor, adding in your butter, heavy cream and cheese. Puree until whipped, seasoning with sea salt and black pepper.

Nutrition Facts:

Calories: 183

Fat: 15 Grams

Net Carbs: 4 Grams

Protein: 8 Grams

Creamy Spinach

Serves: 4
Time: 40 Minutes
Ingredients:

- 1 Tablespoon Butter
- ½ Sweet Onion, Sliced Thin
- ¾ Cup Heavy Whipping Cream
- 4 Cups Spinach, Torn
- ¼ Cup Herbed Chicken Stock
- Pinch Nutmeg
- Sea Salt & Black Pepper to Taste

Directions:

1. Melt your butter in a skillet over medium heat, and then add in your onion. Cook until lightly caramelized which should take about five minutes.
2. Stir your heavy cream, chicken stock, and spinach in. season with your sea salt, black pepper and nutmeg, stirring again. Sauté until your spinach is wilted, which should take about five minutes.
3. Cook until your spinach is tender and your sauce has thickened, which should take about fifteen minutes.
4. Serve warm.

Nutrition Facts:
Calories: 195
Fat: 20 Grams
Net Carbs: 1 Grams
Protein: 3 Grams

Crisp Zucchini

Serves: 4

Time: 25 Minutes

Ingredients:

- 2 Tablespoons Butter
- 4 Zucchini, Cut into ¼ Inch Rounds
- Black Pepper to Taste
- ½ Cup Parmesan Cheese, Grated

Directions:

1. Start by placing your butter in a skillet over medium-high heat.
2. Once your butter is melted, then add in your zucchini. Cook until tender and lightly brown, which should take about five minutes.
3. Spread your zucchini evenly, sprinkling your parmesan over it.
4. Cook until your parmesan melts, which should take about five minutes.
5. Serve immediately.

Nutrition Facts:

Calories: 94

Fat: 8 Grams

Net Carbs: 1 Grams

Protein: 4 Grams

Zucchini Noodles with Pesto

Serves: 4
Time: 15 Minutes
Ingredients:

- 4 Zucchini, Small & Ends Trimmed
- ¾ Cup Kale Pesto, Keto Friendly
- ¼ Cup Parmesan, Grated

Directions:

1. Start by spiralizing your zucchini, and then add in your pesto.
2. Top with parmesan before serving chilled.

Nutrition Facts:
Calories: 93
Fat: 8 Grams
Net Carbs: 2 Grams
Protein: 4 Grams

Asparagus with Walnuts

Serves: 4
Time: 15 Minutes
Ingredients:

- 1 ½ Tablespoons Olive Oil
- ¾ lb. Asparagus, Trimmed
- Sea Salt & Black Pepper to Taste
- ¼ Cup Walnuts, Chopped

Directions:

1. Start by placing your skillet over medium-high heat. Add in your olive oil.
2. Once your olive oil is hot, add in your asparagus. Cook for five minutes. They should become tender and lightly browned.
3. Season with salt and pepper, and then toss with walnuts before serving.

Nutrition Facts:
Calories: 124
Fat: 12 Grams
Net Carbs: 2 Grams
Protein: 3 Grams

Conclusion

The ketogenic diet is perfect if you want to improve your health and shed those extra pounds. Now that you've finished this book, you should know everything you need to start your ketogenic journey. Not only will you lose weight, but you can reap other benefits such as your blood sugar and blood pressure being reduced, your cholesterol will be improved, and much more. Thank you for downloading this book, and I wish you the best with your keto lifestyle!

Made in the USA
Columbia, SC
18 September 2018